Get Rid Of Bad Breath Once And For All

Leave The Nightmare Behind You

By

Natalie Johnson

Table of Contents

Introduction

I want to thank you and congratulate you for purchasing the book, "Get Rid Bad Breath Once and for All".

This book contains proven steps and strategies on how to treat bad breath, which will not only boost your self-esteem but will also help you avoid other illnesses associated with halitosis.

In here, the different causes of bad breath are explored, including illnesses and intake of certain kinds of food. The classifications of breath according to its smell are also presented along with the methods for diagnosis—both self and professional diagnosis.

Thanks again for purchasing this book, I hope you enjoy it!

Chapter 1:

The Vulgar Traitor that is Halitosis

If you have rushed into a marriage and your wife is a Jew, and you wanted out, here is a quick fix for you: find out if your wife has foul breath and divorce her. According to a text called Talmud where Jewish laws and customs are based, bad breath is thought to be a serious disability and a husband who finds out that his wife has it could cancel the ketuba, or the marriage contract, over it. Bad breath, also known as halitosis, though, is a serious condition that affects 35-45% of the world population in ways more than just meddle with their marriage. Although a serious case of it could extinguish the fires of romance, a bad breath is not only an indication of a poor oral hygiene but a good indicator of other underlying diseases, as well, such as diabetes, Sjögren's syndrome, xerostomia and chronic bronchitis, among others.

The issue of resolving bad breath with urgency is compelling not just because of the social discomfort it causes but because, as it is primarily caused by periodontal disease brought about by poor oral hygiene, it is correlated to coronary artery disease (commonly called heart disease) which kills approximately 600,000 people in the United States every year. Remarkably, though, experts are beginning to see the preventive benefits of ensuring and maintaining a perfect oral health to avert heart disease; and there is no better way to assess oral health than through our breaths.

Your Bad Breath can Kill Your Heart

When a person does not observe proper oral care as flossing and brushing, the bacteria normally present in the mouth proliferate and feed on left-over food debris in between the teeth, in plaques, in the gums and in the coating at the back of the tongue. After feeding off left-over food particles and dead cells in the mouth, these bacteria produce a smelly gas which is the primary cause of the bad breath.

Some researchers speculate that at a certain point in time during a periodontal disease, bacteria from the mouth and gums enter the bloodstream which set off an immune response similar to inflammation. Scientists believe that, with or without an infection, an inflammation increases the likelihood of blood clot formation. Clots are known to decrease blood flow to the heart, hence an insufficient oxygen supply. This consequently prompts it to overwork to compensate for the said deficiency thereby increasing blood pressure and the risk of heart attack.

Disadvantages of Having a Bad Breath

Just as how you look can tell more things about your personality, so can how your breath smells.

The American Dental Association (ADA) estimates that more than 80 million people in the US alone have chronic halitosis (persistent bad breath). As common as it is, afflicting 1 in every four Americans, it greatly affects sufferers in many ways that they spend over $10 billion each year on oral hygiene products just to combat it.

Here are the bad sides of having halitosis:

- **Bad breath ruins any chance for relationships.** As most intimate relationship involves kissing, a foul breath would make this activity unenjoyable. Recurrent and persistent bad breath will ultimately discourage a partner from pursuing a relationship. This is confirmed by a survey conducted by Match.com involving 5,000 singles of which 2,150 participants listed fresh breath as a foremost consideration to agree to a date and which placed halitosis to the top 3 most unattractive traits in a mate. Those who have foul breaths are known to have fewer partner prospects, dates less often and have lower chances of getting laid.

- **Bad breath lowers self-esteem.** As sufferers begin to notice people avoiding a conversation with them or passing hurtful remarks about the smell of their breaths, lowering of their self-esteem soon follows inevitably. This could lead to anxiety, depression and stress, could cause problems with friendships and romantic relationships and could be a reason for decreased academic and job performance, which ultimately adds up to the further lowering of their self-esteem.

- **Bad breath is correlated to lower income.** A study reveals that those who have chronic halitosis tend to belong to the group of those who earn less and struggle with promotion. This is because bad breath negatively impacts the impression on your personality and your job opportunity. The Australian Breath Clinic warns that with job conditions being more competitive and with employers becoming increasingly selective, people who work in customer service or those who face customers are more likely to be fired if they do not meet a strict set of requirements, including that which ensures them to have fresh breath.

Three Types of Odors Associated with Bad Breath

The odor of the mouth with halitosis is classified into three groups based on their quality:

- **Sulfurous or fecal breath.** It is estimated that 85 to 90% of those who suffer from halitosis has this characteristic odor brought about by the presence of volatile sulfur compounds, which are waste products produced by oral bacteria as they feed off dead cells and food particles left inside the mouth, in between teeth, in the gums and at the back of the tongue. These compounds produce odors like rotten egg (hydrogen sulfide), barnyard (methyl mercaptan) and a smelly ocean (dimethyl sulfide). In addition to volatile sulfur compounds, these bacteria give off other compounds as well such as putrescine (smells like a rotten meat), isovaleric acid (smells like sweaty feet), skatole (smells like a human poop), and cadaverine (smells like a dead animal).

- **Fruity breath.** Halitosis with this type of odor is caused by another condition not found inside the mouth: diabetes. People who have diabetes have difficulty acquiring energy from blood sugar. Because of this, the body resorts to getting energy by burning stored fat. The breakdown of fats results in the production of a class of compounds known as ketone bodies (or simply ketones). One of which has a characteristic fruity smell called acetone. People who have acetone in their blood have a fruity-smelling breath which smells like nail polish (since a nail polish is basically acetone).

- **Ammoniacal or urine-like breath.** Kidney failure and a disease associated with the failure of the body to metabolize trimethylamine (TMA) properly cause a particular type of halitosis characterized by strong urine-like and fishy odors as a result of the buildup of nitrogenous waste products in the blood such as ammonia, dimethyl amine and trimethylamine.

Chapter 2:

What Causes Bad Breath?

Halitosis or bad breath cannot be singled out as a simple disease of the mouth. Although its primary cause is the negligence in oral hygiene resulting in oral infection and bacterial conditions that produce foul gases, sometimes the cause of a smelly odor emanating through the breath is a complex chemical-based dysfunction inside the body associated with more serious illnesses. Here are the causes of bad breath:

- **Bacteria.** There are about 75 to 100 different kinds of bacteria that live in a person's mouth. Some of which protect against foul breath and are considered good while some causes the malodor associated with halitosis. Normally, the bacteria that cause bad odor live in the teeth and in plaque but are more concentrated at the back of the mouth. The moist and warm condition inside the mouth and the accumulation of food particles at the back of the mouth cause these types of bacteria to proliferate. While they feed off dead cells and food particles, they give off compounds made of sulfur that gives the unpleasant odor of halitosis. A new research conducted in Japan found out that the very bacteria associated with bad breath are those which cause stomach ulcer and cancer, as well.

- **Empty stomach in the morning.** During sleep, the mouth is under less activity and saliva content as with waking hours. This sudden change in the condition inside the mouth favors the multiplication of these organisms responsible for bad breath. Eating breakfast stimulates the production of saliva which, along with the food-swallowing process, scrapes off and flushes out the bacteria at the back of the tongue that causes foul breath. Without these, bacteria are left to grow and produce sulfurous compounds. This explains why skipping breakfast equates to bad breath.

- **Medications.** Medications such as antidepressants, aspirin and diuretics can cause a decrease in the production of saliva. Without a sufficient amount of saliva, bacteria are not flushed out of the mouth and are left to multiply and give off bad odor as they feed inside our mouth.

- **Diet.** There are foods that could cause halitosis in multiple different ways. Some cause bad breath through the compound they contain while some cause it by providing more food for the bacteria. Here are the foods t cause halitosis:

- *Onions and garlic.* These spices contain sulfur compounds that, when ingested, are absorbed in the bloodstream. These sulfur compounds, like that which are produced by the bacteria inside our mouth, are expelled through sweat, urine and through the lungs in the form of breath and give off an unpleasant smell.

- *Alcohol and coffee.* These two compounds, alcohol and caffeine, are known to have a drying effect which causes a reduction in the saliva production. It has been explained earlier that reduction of saliva inside the mouth causes an increase in the bacterial content of mouth that consequently leads to foul breath. Furthermore, less saliva means more concentrated volatile compounds and stronger breath odor.

- *Sweet foods.* The bacteria that cause plaque buildup and produce strong odors thrive in the presence of sugar as it provides them a quick source of food and energy enabling them to reproduce exponentially. To avoid this effect, if you are to consume foods rich in sugar, it is advised that you should brush your teeth and scrape your tongue afterwards or at least perform mouth rinse.

- *Acidic Foods.* Acidity is measured in pH. The neutral pH is 7; foods that have a lower pH level than it are considered acidic and those with higher are considered basic. At any time, mouth maintains a normal pH of 6.5 (slightly acidic). Consumption of foods that have lower pH (acidic) increases the acidity of the mouth and encourages the increase in bad bacteria, which favors an acidic environment. These bacteria thrive well in acidic environment and reproduce quickly causing a foul breath in no time.

o ***Low carbohydrate diets.*** A diet that is low in calories from carbohydrates triggers a response from the body to utilize the stored fats for energy. This process results in the production of ketone bodies which include acetone. This compound is highly volatile and is expelled through breath which causes halitosis characterized by a fruity smell.

• **Breathing through the mouth.** Anything that dries the mouth could cause or potentially aggravate an existing halitosis because of two reasons. First, saliva helps wash away dead cells and particles of food. Without enough saliva in the mouth, bacteria tend to multiply because of the abundance of their source of energy. Secondly, saliva dilutes the foul-smelling volatile sulfur compounds and makes them less noticeable. Without enough saliva, these compounds become concentrated and the smell associated with them increases in intensity.

- **Existing illnesses and other medical conditions.** Sometimes, halitosis is an indication of a far more serious condition other than that which concerns oral issues. Here is a list of some of the illnesses that could cause your breath to smell:

o ***Sinus Infection.*** Normally, the sinuses contain only air. Bacterial and/or viral infection of the sinuses triggers an inflammatory response from the immune system which causes the formation of yellowish or greenish mucus-like substance, which is actually a combination of mucus, white blood cells and the volatile compounds which are excreted by bacteria as a waste product (the root cause of the smell). In postnasal drip, or in a condition in which the mucus flows down to the throat, the smell of these substances mix with the breath making it foul and repulsively obnoxious.

o ***Thrush.*** Oral thrush, also known as candidiasis, is a yeast infection caused by the overgrowth of a fungus known as candida. Normally, candida is present in small amounts in the mouth, skin and digestive tract. However, certain medications or medical conditions somehow cause this fungus to proliferate resulting in an infection characterized by the presence of a creamy white and slightly raised lesion in the tongue or at the site of infection. The lesion my resemble a cottage cheese and brushing or scraping them results to pain and bleeding. This characteristic appearance emits a smell that mixes with the breath causing halitosis.

o **Cavities.** Cavities are formed when a certain kind of bacteria known as Streptococcus mutans (or S. mutans) produce acid as a byproduct of metabolizing sugar. This acid eats away the enamel of the teeth and causes tooth decay which forms cavities later. Decayed tooth and cavities give off a foul smell and cause halitosis. A suitable treatment for cavities and tooth decay effectively restores fresh breath.

o *Tonsilolliths.* When bits of food get stuck in the craters of the tonsil, a foul-smelling lump called tonsil stones (or tonsilolliths) are formed composed of the food particle, mucus from postnasal drip and dead cells. Combined with the volatile sulfur compounds produced by the bacteria at the surface of the tongue, tonsil stones could give off a potent repulsive smell that mixes with the breath.

o *Diabetes (Type 1 and Type 2).* Diabetes is thought to cause halitosis in two ways. First, the unstable amount of blood sugar, caused by the body's inability to produce enough insulin or to respond to it effectively, is thought to increase the person's likelihood of contracting gum disease, which is the most common cause of halitosis. Second, since diabetics are unable to utilize sugar as energy, the body resorts to stored fats for energy; the breakdown of which produces ketone bodies, which include acetone that is given off in the lungs and mixes with breath causing a halitosis with a distinctive fruity smell.

- **Cigarette smoking.** In a study conducted and published in 1968 by the journal Chemical Reviews, it was identified that a tobacco contains more than 60 aromatic hydrocarbons; most of which have notable scents. These compounds along with smoke particles stick to and are left at the throat and lungs which are given off in the breath minutes or hours after smoking a cigarette causing a special type of halitosis known as "smoker's breath." In addition, smoking cigarettes dries the mouth creating a favorable condition for the proliferation of the anaerobic bacteria inside the mouth that produces volatile sulfur compounds.

Chapter 3:

How is Bad Breath Diagnosed?

Interestingly, it is virtually impossible for people to smell their own breaths. This is because of a process called habituation in which the brain tends to ignore the scent of our breath because of our constant exposure to it. This is an energy-saving mechanism which enables our brains to focus on more important stimulus. That explains why it is almost impossible, at certain levels of halitosis, for us to perform a self-diagnosis for its presence. However, there are ways to detect the presence of bad breath.

Self-Diagnosis

Here's a list of things that you can perform to test for the presence of halitosis.

- **Lick your wrist.** One simple way to diagnose bad breath is to lick the wrist, wait for about 5 seconds and smell it. The smell from the wrist will tell something about your breath. If it smells foul, then you most certainly have a bad breath. If it smells just like a dried saliva, it means you are free from this embarrassing condition.

- **Cover your nose and mouth with both your palm and breathe.** This method will introduce an increased amount of molecules from your mouth to your olfactory nerves. Doing this will amplify the smell of your breath, which will enable you to smell it.

- **Pull your cheeks back and forth.** Doing this will expose the side of your mouth, which is also one of the places in your mouth that bacteria dwell in the most, revealing any hidden scents within due to the accumulation of volatile sulfur compounds. The smell produced by pulling your cheeks back and forth represents the smell of your breath as perceived by others.

- **Scrape the back of your tongue with a spoon and smell it.** Since the back of your tongue is one of the areas in your mouth which receives the least attention, it is likely that bacteria that cause halitosis thrive in it while avoiding being noticed. The smell of the back of your tongue determines the smell of your breath.

Professional Diagnosis

Here is the list of the methods used by professionals to diagnose halitosis:

- **Halimeter.** This device works by detecting and measuring the amount of a sulfur compound known as hydrogen sulfide in the air inside the mouth. Although this device can effectively detect the presence of bacteria that produces volatile sulfur compounds, results could be unreliable at times since the concentration of sulfur in the mouth air could also be increased by eating certain kinds of food such as garlic and onions.

- **BANA test.** Benzoyl-DL-Argining NaphthylAmide (BANA) test is used to detect the presence of three types of bacteria associated with periodontal disease—one of the major causes of halitosis. This test works by using a compound called BANA, which is known to react with the enzyme possessed by these bacteria. The presence of a reaction indicates the presence of these bacteria, hence, the detection of halitosis.

- **Gas Chromatography.** This test works by detecting the concentration of three major volatile sulfur compounds (namely hydrogen sulfide, dimethyl sulfide and methyl mercaptan) in a sample of air taken inside the mouth. Compared to Halimeter, which somehow works similarly, this technique is considered to be more accurate and provides a visualization of the concentration of the above-mentioned VSCs through a graph displayed in a computer.

- **β-galactosidase test.** In this test concentration of a compound known as β-galactosidase is measured. Studies have revealed that elevated levels of this compound is correlated with bad breath.

Chapter 4:

Treatments for Halitosis

The best way to treat bad breath is to target its cause. Temporary remedies such as using mouthwash and mouth sprays may only do so much to mask the malodor of your mouth, but will do nothing to cure it to its source. Another cause of action, which may not be as permanent, is to neutralize the volatile compounds that cause the odor. A better way, however, is to find the source and the cause of the production of these compounds and stop it at that.

- **Use of antimicrobial toothpastes and mouthwashes.** One of the ways to treat halitosis, if its root cause is an oral problem, is to kill the bacteria that produce the compounds that cause bad breath through the use of antimicrobial oral products. Here are a list of compounds that you should check in oral care products, which kill bacteria by directly acting upon them or by changing the pH of the mouth thereby making the environment unsuitable for them.

- o **Triclosan.** In a review conducted by the FDA on 1997 on the effect of adding triclosan in Colgate Total Toothpaste, they found out the inclusion of it in the said toothpaste decreased the likelihood of contracting periodontal disease. This is because triclosan is known to kill bactcria inside the mouth that does not only cause periodontitis but also halitosis.

- o **Bicarbonate of soda.** Alternatively known as baking soda, this major component of a toothpaste interferes with plaque metabolism and modifies the pH of the mouth thereby making the insides of the mouth a little less favorable environment for bacterial growth.

o **Zinc salts.** Known to have antimicrobial properties, this compound inhibits enzymatic reactions in bacteria particularly that which converts sugar into plaque acid. Zinc ions are also known to have a strong affinity for sulfur compounds and converts them from being volatile to a non-volatile state.

o **Chlorhexidine salts.** These compounds inhibit the production of plaque acid and has antimicrobial properties.

• **Tonsillectomy.** One of the causes of bad breath, which is unknown to most people, is the presence of tonsil stones or tonsilloliths. Tonsil stones have a distinctive fecal odor and are strongly expressed in breath. Halitosis associated with this is best treated by preventing the recurrent formation of tonsilloliths through the removal of the tonsil in a surgical process called a tonsillectomy. People, whose halitosis is caused by persistent formation of tonsilloliths, found their fresh breath restored after this simple operation.

- **Treatment for any underlying illnesses that causes halitosis.** There are multiple conditions that could cause halitosis, which include infection of the sinuses and upper respiratory tract, diabetes and kidney failure. The best way to treat the halitosis that is associated with them is to take the appropriate courses of treatment for those.

- **Removal of decayed tooth and treatment for cavities.** Since rotten teeth are known for their foul odor, and since the presence of tooth decay and cavities causes halitosis, having the decayed teeth removed and the cavities dealt with minimizes, or to some extent, cures halitosis.

- **Improvement in oral hygiene.** An important factor in treating and avoiding halitosis is the maintenance of a healthy oral hygiene. Good oral hygiene greatly reduces the chance for halitosis due to its ability to control the bacterial population inside the mouth. This, in turn, results to diminished chance for tooth decay and tonsillolith formation and a fresher breath.

  o *Brush and floss your teeth every after meal.* Doing this ensures that no food particles are left in the mouth and even in between teeth thereby providing no energy source for bacteria and preventing their proliferation in the mouth.

o ***Clean your tongue with a scraper.*** Dentists advise to scrape your tongue for at least twice a day every day. Recent studies reveal that the cause of halitosis is more likely to be located at the back of the tongue than in teeth and gums.

- **Observance of moderation in alcohol and caffeine intake.** Not only alcohol and caffeine but anything that dries the mouth should be taken with caution and moderation but any other substances that do so because a dry mouth encourages these bacteria to multiply. If, however, consumption of these substances is inevitable, it is therefore imperative that one should take water for hydration to flush away bacteria and food debris and to keep the mouth moist.

Chapter 5:

Healthy Habits of a Halitosis-Free Person

Bad breath is not a condition that you just get overnight. It is the result of a prolonged disregard for oral health, which leads to various conditions of the mouth that results in halitosis. Here are the habits in order to keep bad breath away:

- **Pay a regular visit to your dentist.** No one is more adept at assessing your oral health and providing treatment for whatever illness it has than your dentist. The American Dental Association advises that you pay a visit to your dentist every six months. Almost half the adult population in the US fail to do this because of fear or plain neglect.

- **Avoid or minimize sugary foods.** Sugar supports bad breath in two ways. First, it provides food for the bacteria which give off plaque (the cause of tooth decay) and volatile sulfur compounds that add an array of unpleasant smell in the breath. S it affects the pH of the mouth which further encourages the bacteria to grow and multiply.

- **Stop smoking.** Smoking is a major contributor to halitosis. In order to cure halitosis, one must not only minimize but stop smoking altogether. A cigarette smoke is known to have as many as 60 compounds that have a strong odor. These compounds along with smoke particles stick to the side of the throat and lungs and are given off through the breath hours after smoking.

- **Minimize caffeine intake.** Not only that caffeine acts as mild diuretic and causes dry mouth, it also has a characteristic odor which sticks at the back of the tongue and is expressed through breath. One must consider alternatives to coffee such as herbal or green tea to minimize caffeine-induced halitosis.

Conclusion

Thank you again for purchasing this book!

I hope this book was able to help you to solve your problems with your bad breath. With the tips in this book, you can now confidently socialize and perform your job without having to worry about the smell of your breath.

The next step is to ensure that the factors that cause or aggravate existing halitosis are avoided. You should maintain a healthy oral hygiene too, and make it a point to pay regular visits to your dentist.

If you information in this book was helpful to you, I invite you to leave a review on Amazon. Thanks.

Published by MCJ Publishing:
www.book-o-rama.com

www.ingramcontent.com/pod-product-compliance
Lightning Source LLC
Chambersburg PA
CBHW062026280526
45787CB00005B/2227